101 Healing Bible verses

101 Healing Bible verses

Ed Chatelier

CONTENTS

2 Psalm 146:8

The Lord gives sight to the blind, the Lord lifts up those who are bowed down, the Lord loves the righteous.

If you need healing learn the Bible verses.

Philippians 4:7

God's peace which transcends all understanding, shall garrison and mount guard over my heart and mind in Christ.

Luke 8:50

Hearing this, Jesus said to Jairus, "Don't be afraid; just believe, and she will be healed.

Psalm 146:8

T he Lord gives sight to the blind, the Lord lifts up those who are bowed down, the Lord loves the righteous.

Isaiah 53:5

By his stripes you are healed.

Matthew 8:8

Just say the word and you will be healed.

James 5:16

Therefore, confess your sins to one another and pray for one another, that you may be healed. The prayer of a righteous person has great power as it is working.

John 15:7

I f you abide in me, and my words abide in you, ask whatever you wish, and it will be done for you.

John 6:35

I am the Bread of Life. I give you life.

Isaiah 54:17

No weapon forged against you will prevail, and you will refute every tongue that accuses you. This is the heritage of the servants of the Lord, and this is their vindication from me," declares the Lord.

Acts 4:30

I stretch forth My hand to heal.

1 Peter 1:3

Praise be to the God and Father of our Lord Jesus Christ! In his great mercy he has given us new birth into a living hope through the resurrection of Jesus Christ from the dead.

Revelation 21:4

And God will wipe away every tear from their eyes; there shall be no more death, nor sorrow, nor crying. There shall be no more pain, for the former things have passed away.

Psalm 147:3

The Lord heals the broken hearted and binds up their wounds.

Acts 9:34

I, Jesus Christ make you whole.

Acts 3:16

Faith in My Name makes you strong and gives you perfect sound-ness.

16

Luke 9:56

I am not come to destroy men's lives but to save them.

Acts 19:12

My power causes diseases to depart from you.

Romans 8:2

The law of the spirit of life in Me has made you free from the law of sin and death.

John 8:32

A nd you will know the truth, and the truth will set you free.

2 Coriinthians 1:10

I have delivered you from death, I do deliver you, and if you trust Me, I will yet deliver you.

2 Corinthians 4:11

My life may be manifest in your mortal flesh.

Philippians 4:6-7

I will not fret or have anxiety about anything, but in every circumstance and in everything, by prayer and petition, with thanksgiving, continue to make my requests known to God.

Hebrews 12:12,13

Lift up the weak hands and feeble knees; don't let that which is lame be turned aside but rather let Me heal it.

Matthew 9:35

A nd Jesus went throughout all the cities and villages, teaching in their synagogues and proclaiming the gospel of the kingdom and healing every disease and every affliction.

Romans 5:3-4

"Not only that, but we rejoice in our sufferings, knowing that suffering produces endurance, and endurance produces character, and character produces hope..."

Luke 10:19

Behold, I give you authority over all the enemy's power and nothing shall by any means hurt you.

Mark 9:23

If you can believe, all things are possible to him that believes.

Isaiah 40:29-31

In my weakness, He increases strength in me. I wait for Him [expect, look for and hope in Him] and He renews my strength and power. I will lift up with wings of strength and rise as an eagle. I shall run and not be weary, I shall walk and not faint or become tired.

Isaiah 32:3, 35:5

The eyes of the blind shall be opened; the eyes of them that see shall not be dim. The ears of the deaf shall be unstopped; the ears of them that hear shall hearken.

3 John 1:2

"**D**ear friend, I pray that you may enjoy good health and that all may go well with you, even as your soul is getting along well."

Matthew 8:3

I will, be thou clean.

Isaiah 38:16,20

I will recover you and make you to live; I am ready to save you.

33

James 5:14,15

Is anyone among you sick? Let him call for the elders of the church, and let them pray over him, anointing him with oil in the name of the Lord.

Ezekiel 34:16

I will bind up that which was broken and will strengthen that which was sick.

Isaiah 53:5

He was wounded for your transgressions.
   He was bruised for our iniquities.
   The punishing of our peace is upon him.
   By his stripes you are healed.

Psalm 103

Who crowns you with steadfast love and mercy, who satisfies you with good so that your youth is renewed like the eagle's.

Philippians 1:6

I am convinced and sure that He who began a good work in me will continue until the day of Jesus Christ, developing and perfecting and bringing it to full completion in me.

Isaiah 58:8

Your light shall break forth as the morning and your health shall spring forth speedily.

Matthew 8:13

Then Jesus said to the centurion, 'Go! Let it be done just as you believed it would.' And his servant was healed at that moment.

Isaiah 57:18-19

I Have Seen Their Ways, But I Will Heal Them; I Will Guide Them And Restore Comfort To Israel's Mourners, Creating Praise On Their Lips. Peace, Peace, To Those Far And Near,' Says The Lord, 'And I Will Heal Them.'"

John 14:27

Peace I leave with you; my peace I give you. I do not give to you as the world gives. Do not let your hearts be troubled and do not be afraid.

Isaiah 32:4

The tongue of the dumb shall sing;

Proverbs 16:24

My pleasant Words are sweet to your soul and health to your bones.

Philippians 4:13

I can do all things through him who strengthens me.

Isaiah 41:10

Fear not, for I am with you; be not dismayed, for I am your God; I will strengthen you, I will help you, I will uphold you with my righteous right hand.

Isaiah 53:5

"But he was pierced for our transgressions, he was crushed for our iniquities; the punishment that brought us peace was on him, and by his wounds we are healed."

Proverbs 4:20-22

My son, be attentive to my words; incline your ear to my sayings. Let them not escape from your sight; keep them within your heart. For they are life to those who find them, and healing to all their flesh.

4:22

My Words are life to you, and health and medicine to all your flesh.

Psalm 91:14

B ecause I have set my love on the Lord, therefore He delivers me.
He sets me securely on high, because I have known His Name.

Luke 6:19

"And the people all tried to touch him, because power was coming from him and healing them all."

Proverbs 17:52

A cheerful heart is good medicine, but a crushed spirit dries up the bones.

Acts 10:38

I do good and heal all that are oppressed of the devil.

Amos 5:4,6

S eek Me and you shall live.

Malachi 4:2

I have arisen with healing in My wings.

Deuteronomy 33:25

As your days, so shall your strength be.

Deuteronomy 7:15

And the Lord will take away from you all sickness, and none of the evil diseases of Egypt, which you knew, will he inflict on you, but he will lay them on all who hate you.

Matthew 4:23

I heal all manner of sickness and all manner of disease.

Luke 14:8

The Spirit of the Lord is on me, because he has anointed me to proclaim good news to the poor. He has sent me to proclaim freedom for the prisoners and recovery of sight for the blind, to set the oppressed free.

Matthew 14:14

I am moved with compassion toward the sick and I heal them.

Matthew 9:29

A ccording to your faith, be it unto you.

Proverbs 4:10

The years of your life shall be many.

Deuteronomy 23:5

I turned the curse into a blessing unto you because I love you.

Deuteronomy 11:9-21

It will be well with you and your days shall be multiplied and prolonged as the days of heaven upon earth.

2 Kings 20:5

Go Back And Tell Hezekiah, The Ruler Of My People, 'This Is What The Lord, The God Of Your Father David, Says: I Have Heard Your Prayer And Seen Your Tears; I Will Heal You. On The Third Day From Now You Will Go Up To The Temple Of The Lord.'

Deuteronomy 32:39

See now that I, even I, am he, and there is no god with me: I kill, and I make alive; I wound, and I heal: neither is there any that can deliver out of my hand.

Deuteronomy 28:61

I have redeemed you from every sickness and every plague.

Isaiah 53:4

I bore your sickness.

Matthew 8:17

I took your infirmities. I bore your sickness.

Matthew 9:12

If you're sick you need a physician. I am the Lord your physician.

2 Corinthians 10:3-5

Even though I have a physical body, I will not carry on warfare according to the flesh, using mere human weapons. The weapons of my warfare are not physical (weapons of flesh and blood), they are mighty before God for the overthrow and destruction of strongholds. I refute arguments and theories and reasonings and every proud and lofty thing that sets itself up against the true knowledge of God; and I lead every thought and purpose away captive into the obedience of Christ.

Psalm 30: 2

I have healed you and brought up your soul from the grave;

2 Corinthians 12:9

But he said to me, 'My grace is sufficient for you, for my power is made perfect in weakness.' Therefore I will boast all the more gladly of my weaknesses, so that Christ's power may rest on me."

2 Chronicles 17:14

If my people, who are called by my name, will humble themselves and pray and seek my face and turn from their wicked ways, then I will hear from heaven, and I will forgive their sin and will heal their land.

Exodus 15:26

I am the Lord that healeth thee.

Psalm 107:20

He sent his word and it healed them.

75

Psalm 73:26

My flesh and my heart may fail, but God is the strength of my heart and my portion forever.

Psalm 103:3

I heal all your diseases.

Ezekiel 37:5,14

Behold, I will cause breath to enter into you and you shall live; and I shall put My Spirit in you and you shall live.

John 10:10

The thief comes only to steal and kill and destroy. The Lord came that I may have and enjoy life, and have it in abundance (to the full, till it overflows).

I am the resurrection and the life.

John 14:14

I f you ask anything in My name, I will do it.

Romans 8:11

The same Spirit that raised Me from the dead now lives in you and that Spirit will quicken your mortal body.

Romans 8:1

There is therefore now no condemnation for those who are in Christ Jesus.

Isaiah 40:29

He giveth power to the faint; and to them that have no might he increaseth strength.

1 Corinthians 6:19-20

Your body is the temple of My Spirit and you are to glorify Me in your body.

Matthew 15:30

"**G**reat crowds came to him, bringing the lame, the blind, the crippled, the mute and many others, and laid them at his feet; and he healed them."

Psalm 41:4

I said, Lord, be merciful unto me: heal my soul; for I have sinned against thee.

Numbers 12:13

A nd Moses cried unto the Lord, saying, Heal her now, O God, I beseech thee.

Isaiah 46:4

To your old age and gray hairs I will carry you. and I will deliver you.

Colossians 1:13

I have delivered you from the authority of darkness.

I Corinthians 12:9

I have sent gifts of healing in My Body.

1 Corinthians 10:13

No temptation has overtaken you that is not common to man. God is faithful, and he will not let you be tempted beyond your ability, but with the temptation he will also provide the way of escape, that you may be able to endure it.

Isaiah 53

S urely he bears your sicknesses and carries your diseases.

Genesis 6:3

Your days shall be one hundred and twenty years.

Psalm 29:11

I will give you strength and bless you with peace.

Nehimiah 8:10

My joy is your strength. A merry heart does good like a medicine.

Exodus 12:13

When I see the blood, I will pass over you, and the plague shall not be upon you to destroy you.

James 5:15

A nd the prayer of faith will save the one who is sick, and the Lord will raise him up. And if he has committed sins, he will be forgiven.

John 1:4

In Me is life.

Philippians 4:19

And my God will meet all your needs according to the riches of his glory in Christ Jesus.

2 Timothy 4:18

I will deliver you from every evil work.

Exodus 15:26

Saying, "If you will diligently listen to the voice of the Lord your God, and do that which is right in his eyes, and give ear to his commandments and keep all his statutes, I will put none of the diseases on you that I put on the Egyptians, for I am the Lord, your healer."

Exodus 23: 26

I will take sickness away from the midst of you and the number of your days I will fulfil.

Psalm 6:2

Be gracious to me, O Lord, for I am languishing; heal me, O Lord, for my bones are troubled.

Psalm 30:2

L ORD my God, I called to you for help, and you healed me."

Psalm 91:16

I call upon the Lord, and He answers me. God is with me in trouble. He delivers and honors me. With long life He will satisfy me and show me His salvation.

Psalm 103:1-5

B less the Lord, O my soul, and forget not all his benefits, who for-
gives all your sins(iniquity), who heals all your diseases, who re-
deems your life from the pit,

Hosea 6:1

"Come, let us return to the Lord.
For He has torn us, but He will heal us;
He has wounded us, but He will bandage us."

Matthew 4:23

A nd he went through out all Galilee, teaching in their synagogues and proclaiming the gospel of the kingdom and healing every disease and every affliction among the people.

Ezekiel 47:9

Every living thing where the rivers goes, will live; for they will be healed, and everything will live wherever the river goes.

Matthew 8:1-3

When Jesus Came Down From The Mountainside, Large Crowds Followed Him. A Man With Leprosy Came And Knelt Before Him

And Said, "Lord, If You Are Willing, You Can Make Me Clean." Jesus Reached Out His Hand And Touched The Man. "I Am Willing," He Said. "Be Clean!" Immediately He Was Cleansed Of His Leprosy.

John 6:63

The words I speak unto you are spirit and life.

1 Peter 2:24

"'He Himself bore our sins' in His body on the cross, so that we might die to sins and live for righteousness; 'by His wounds you have been healed.'"

Isaiah 53:5

With My wounds you are healed.

Genesis 15:15

You shall be buried in a good old age (Gen 15:15)

Isaiah 57:10

I carried your pains.

Psalm 41:2,3

I will preserve you and keep you alive.
The Lord sustains him on his sickbed; in his illness you restore him to full health.

Psalm 91:9-10

Because I have made the Lord my refuge, and the Most High my dwelling place, there shall no evil befall me, nor any plague or calamity come near my house.

Isaiah 33:2

"LORD, be gracious to us; we long for you. Be our strength every morning, our salvation in time of distress."

Isaiah 57:19

I will heal you.

Jeremiah 17:14

Heal me, O Lord, and I shall be healed; save me, and I shall be saved, for you are my praise.

Matthew 4:36

A s many as touch Me are made perfectly whole.

Matthew 15:26

Healing is the children's bread.

Mark 5:34

He said to her, 'Daughter, your faith has healed you. Go in peace and be freed from your suffering.'

Mark 7:37

I do all things well. I make the deaf to hear and the dumb to speak.

Ephesians 6:3

I want it to be well with you and I want you to live long on the earth.

Jeremiah 30:17

But I will restore you to health and heal your wounds,' declares the LORD, 'because you are called an outcast, Zion for whom no one cares.'

Jeremiah 33:6

Behold, I will bring to it health and healing, and I will heal them and reveal to them abundance of prosperity and security.

Proverbs 15:30

(**M**^y) good report makes your bones fat.

Isaiah 35:6

The lame man shall leap as a deer.

Matthew 10:1

And he called to him his twelve disciples and gave them authority over unclean spirits, to cast them out, and to heal every disease and every affliction.

Matthew 12:15

I heal them all.

Matthew 10:8

Heal the sick, raise the dead, cleanse those who have leprosy, drive out demons. Freely you have received; freely give.

Philippians 4:6

Do not be anxious about anything, but in everything by prayer and supplication with thanksgiving let your requests be made known to God.

Isaiah 40:29

"He gives strength to the weary (faint)and increases the power of the weak."

Isaiah 40:31

I will renew your strength I will strengthen and help you.

Proverbs 3:7-8

Be not wise in your own eyes; fear the Lord, and turn away from evil. It will be healing to your flesh and refreshment to your bones.

Mark 10:52

Go," said Jesus, "your faith has healed you." Immediately he received his sight and followed Jesus along the road.

Mark 16:18

When hands are laid on you, you shall recover.

Luke 9:11

I heal all those who have need of healing (Luke9:11)

Hebrews 11:1

Now faith is the assurance of things hoped for, the conviction of things not seen.

2 Timothy 1:7

God has not given me a spirit of timidity and fear. He has given me a spirit of power and of love and of a calm and well-balanced mind, discipline and self-control.

Hebrews 2:9,14,15

I tasted death for you. I destroyed the devil who had the power of death. I've delivered you from the fear of death and bondage.

Ephesians 1:21

I have given you My Name and have put all things under your feet.

1 Corinthians 11:29-31

If you'll rightly discern My body which was broken for you, and judge yourself, you'll not be judged and you'll not be weak, sickly or die prematurely.

1 Corinthians 11:29-31

If you'll rightly discern My body which was broken for you, and judge yourself, you'll not be judged and you'll not be weak, sickly or die prematurely.

Luke 4:18

My anointing delivers the broken-hearted, and delivers the captives, recovers sight to the blind and sets at liberty those that are bruised.

Conclusion

If you have reached the end of this book well done. REMEMBER GOD PRAY DOES HEAL !

Everyone gets ill or knows someone who is ill at sometime. Medical Science can offer healing and some relief but many times diagnosis and cost leaves you coming up short.It is encouraging to know that God of the Bible can heal. This books draws out the key promises of God that can open the Door to your healing. Just read the verses on each page and speak them out. Let the words sink in and I believe you will get peace , comfort and healing. SPEAK OUT , MEDITATE and PRAY and BELIEVE.